Nutrition Meets Neurology

Aries Ford

BS, RDN, LDN

Register Dietitian Nutritionist

Copyright © 2016 Aries Ford

Global Impact Publishing

Winston Salem, NC

AriesFord.org

All rights reserved. No part of this book may be reproduced in any form or by any means, electronic or mechanical including photocopying, recording, or by any information storage and retrieval system without prior written permission of the publisher, excepting brief quotes in connection with medical training.

Printed in the United States of America

*This book is intended as an informative nutritional guide for best practice in the Neuroscience setting. I encourage continued collaboration with a dietitian and other professional team members in neurology. Registered Dietitians are the Nutrition experts that focus to assist the neurology team as well as strive to provide patients with expert quality care.

Table of contents

Chapter 1: Objectives and Overview

Chapter 2: Benefits of Early Feeding Verses Delayed Feeding in ICU

Chapter 3: Indications for Enteral Nutrition Support and Tube Selection

Chapter 4: Energy Expenditure, Mechanical Ventilation and Your Patient

Chapter 5: Typical Considerations for Neurology Enteral Patients

Chapter 6: Indications for Central Nutrition Support (TPN)

Chapter 7: Indications for Peripheral Nutrition Support

Chapter 8: What is Refeeding Syndrome?

Chapter 9: Post Extubation Options

Chapter 10: Success Advantages in Discharge Disposition's

SPECIAL APPRECIATION

To the entire Neurology, Neurosurgical and Radiology team including all disciplines who facilitate compassion, amazing care for their patients and expect healing results.

Introduction

I'd like to take a moment and introduce myself and what sparked my interest in Neurology. I was offered the opportunity to work in Neurology and was met by many interesting cases. I've watched miracles happen as the neurology team worked so closely together unitedly. I developed such a compassion for the patients and wanted to provide the best possible care that I could provide as a dietitian. I wanted to contribute and make a dramatic difference in the lives of the patients and their families. Therefore, I begin to look at areas of concerns, research strategies and the tools to promote better outcomes in regards to nutrition.

My goal is to share the nutritional strategies in reducing length of stay, maintaining nutritional status, minimizing or preventing sarcopenia, preserving lean body mass and getting your patient home as independently as possible.

Chapter 1: Overview of the Annual Neurology Symposium

- To identify Indications for Medical Nutrition Therapy in Neurology and the benefits of early feeding.

- To identify Indications and contraindications of types of nutrition support and feeding access.

- Exploring various options post extubation.

- Discuss risk for suboptimal PO intake and how nutritional supplementation can improve your patients ability to discharge home.

Chapter 2: Benefits of Early Feeding Verses Delayed Feeding in ICU

1. Decreases ICU LOS
2. Decreases ventilator support
3. Better wound healing and reduces risk for sarcopenia
4. Helps preserve GI tract integrity
5. Recommended within 24-48 hours of ICU admission

McClave et al SA, Martindale RG, Vanek VW, et al
Society of Critical Care Medicine (SCCM) and American Society for Parenteral and Enteral Nutrition (ASPEN).JPEN J Parenter/Enteral Nutr.2009:33(3):277-316

Meta-analyses aggregated data suggest
- Reduced mortality when EN was started within 48 hours
- Reduction in infectious morbidity
- Reduction in hospital LOS

Chapter 3: Indications for Nutrition Support and Tube Selection

For those patients who are deemed with any of the following:

1. NPO status
2. Intubation
3. Functioning gut
4. Malnourished and unable to take a full oral diet

*Contraindication-
Non-functioning Gut

Types of Feeding Tubes

- DHT- more comfortable
- OG tube- ventilator patients
- NG tubes- short term support
- PEG- long term support
- J-Tubes

DHT (dobhoff tube) is more comfortable however, medications can clog these tubes easily. Consut with your pharmacist for proper medication administration.

OG (orogastric) tubes typically used for ventilator patients, but not in every case.

NG (nasogastric)tubes for short term support. Hoping the patient will eventually pass a swallow evaluation.

PEG (percutaneous endoscopic) tubes can be placed in the event your patient will need tube feedings for greater than 1 month.

Jejunostomy tubes are placed directly into the small intestines – you may use these with patients who have are diagnosed with pancreatitis or may be considered high risk for aspiration.

Chapter 4: Energy Expenditure, Mechanical Ventilation and your patient

- "Energy expenditure in patients with nontraumatic intracranial hemorrhage"
- <u>JPEN J Parenter Enteral Nutr</u>
  - Intracerebral hemorrhage (ICH)
  - Intraventricular hemorrhage (IVH)
  - Subarachnoid hemorrhage (SAH)
  - Increased morbidity and mortality than other forms of strokes
- Translates to higher nutritional requirements
- <u>Method:</u>
- 14 mechanically hemorrhagic ventilated patients verse 6 severe TBI patients
- 11 out of 14 pt's were sedated

- Glasgow Coma Scale (GCS) scores 4-9
- Indirect Calorimetry Testing (ICT) performed within 7 days of admission
- Average age: 59 years

Most practitioners would assume the nutritional requirements for TBI would be greater than hemorrhagic strokes. We are aware of the hypermetabolic response generated in TBI patients. This particular study performed a retrospective study comparing two cohorts of patients.

The average metabolic needs were very similar in reviewing the ICT test between the two.

- Indirect Calorimetry Testing (ICT)
- Measures O_2 consumed and CO_2 exhaled
- Estimates adequate nutritional support of a critically ill patients
- Nutritional composition altered to meet the

demands of neuro patients

- In summary, favorable outcomes can be achieved as nutritional requirements are met and provided for your neurology patients.

Let's take a look at another interesting study.

The effect of nutritional support on outcome from severe head injury

- Journal of Neurosurgery
- 51 brain injured pt's
- GCS scores 4-10 upon admission

Summary- Early initiation of adequate calories and protein was shown to increase long term favorable outcomes.

The research team at the division of neurosurgery assessed 51 brain injured patients within 24 hours of admission. Initial GCS scores ranged from 4-10.

Nutritional interventions were implemented. These patients were monitored and GCS scores were measured at 3 months, 6 months and one year post injury. GCS scores increased by an average of 4 points in the patients that received increased protein and calories upon admission.

Chapter 5: Typical Considerations for Neurology Enteral Patients

Enteral Nutrition in critical care and in noncritical care settings or medical surgical units as follows:

Neuroscience Critical Care

- Formula selection based on medical status, diagnosis, labs, nutrition history and so on
- Flushes: 30 ml every 4 hours especially in patients who are at risk for cerebral edema
- Continuous feeding regimen recommended to improve tolerance in lieu of reduced bowel motility in some patients
  - Collaboration with the dietitian regarding your patient and your total fluid goals for nutrition

Non Critical care
(Neuro Med Surge)
What typically needs to be considered.
- PEG-Pt may transition to bolus feeds to prepare for discharge home
- Free water flushes adjusted to replace maintenance IVF
- Standard formula for long term use

Chapter 6: Indications for Central Nutrition Support (TPN)

- Bowel obstructions/ Ileus
- Resections or planned resections
- GI hemorrhage
- Fistula output>500 mL
- Inability to obtain enteral access for >7 day
- NPO expected to exceed 5-10 days
- Requires central line access
- Nutrition Support Team or pharmacy consult

*Contraindication- Functioning Gut

- Composition: dextrose, amino acids, lipids, trace elements and electrolytes

- -requires central venous access

- The nutrition support team or metabolic team/pharmacy have the ability to provide adequate nutrition and to manipulate electrolyte composition to improve laboratory values

- Electrolytes and additives may be added in addition to macronutrients (dextrose, amino acids and lipids).

*Such as the following; sodium, potassium, chloride, acetate, phosphorus, magnesium, calcium

- <u>Additives</u>:multivitamins, trace elements, thiamine , folic acid, protonix and insulin

- Composition changes daily to maximize what's best for the patient hemodynamically

- What do we need to know about your neuro patient?

    - Is your pt at risk for cerebral edema? Pt's who are at risk will likely require a hypertonic solution to help with management. At least until swelling improves and the neurologist changes the treatment plan.

    - What else should you discuss with the Dietitian or the team that's managing the pt's TPN ?

- Collaborate with the dietitian regarding the amount of total fluids (IVF plus TPN fluids). Your patient may need a lower volume than the typical patient that requires nutrition support.

- Electrolyte goals especially if your patient is on mannitol or 3% saline. Typical nutrition support goal for serum sodium is ~140. However, patients with cerebral edema may have a short term goal of or as high as 155. The team managing TPN will need to be notified. As well as good blood glucose management. Consult the glycemic management team as needed.

Chapter 7: Indications for Peripheral Nutrition Support

- Requires peripheral access

- NPO status is not expected to exceed 3-5 days

- Neurology patients who may be awaiting follow up swallow evaluations within 24-48 hours

- Provides standard electrolytes and usually not as customized as TPN

- Watch total fluid volume *in pt's with cerebral edema , CHF, renal dz, liver dz.*

- *Lipids -when to add and in what frequency*

Chapter 8: What is refeeding syndrome?

What is it?
How do we prevent and treat it?

- Shifts in fluids and electrolytes that occur in malnourished patients

    - History of poor intake prior to admission or NPO>7 days

    - Profound weight loss

    - Malabsorptive syndrome

    - Oncology or Elderly patients

    - Alcoholism

- Primary biomarkers

    - Hypokalemia, hypomagnesemia, hypophosphatemia

    - Often seen with the initiation of nutrition support

Prevention and Treatment

- **Slow progression of nutrition support for those who are deemed at risk. Avoid overfeeding.**

- **Replace abnormalities and monitor**

- **Add thiamine and folic acid for 5 days or per MD/pharmacist best practice guidelines**

Chapter 9: Post Extubation Options

Some patients continue to experience lethargy post extubation. It's okay to leave the feeding tube in for an extra day until the speech therapist can re-assess.

- Nocturnal feeding regimen- while waiting for a swallow evaluation, this will allow for improved appetite and PO intake during the day. See TF initiation guidelines.

- Oral supplements
    - Determined according to acceptable texture to reduce aspiration risk and medical status/diagnosis/labs

- Offer a variety of palatable options to improve acceptance. Appetites vary and it's likely that dysphagia patients will need additional calories and protein in the event they are not able to meet their metabolic needs at meal time if they are not consuming at least 50-75%

Chapter 10: Success Advantage in Discharge Dispositions

Intensive Nutritional Supplements!

"Can improve outcomes in stroke rehabilitation"

Neurology (aan.com)
- *Poor nutrition is a common complication in stroke patients*

Method/Test: Randanmized
- Nutritional supplements were given to 116 undernourished patients

- Functional Independence Measure (FIM) performed upon admission and at discharge. Patients were given the 2 min & 6 min walk test

- FIM motor sub scores were measured as well as length of stay and discharge disposition

Summary
- Increased scores in FIM and motor
- Increased the number of pt's who

were able to discharge home verses SNF

This study compared outcome measurements of intensive nutrition supplementation verses standard nutritional supplementation in 116 undernourished patients admitted to a stroke service. Comparison example includes 1 commercially available supplement per day compared to 2-3 commercial supplements daily.

<u>How can we help at this facility?</u>

1. Assist patients who require feeding assistance

2. Ensure that nursing staff and CNA's document all food and supplements consumed.

3. Document food consumed from outside of the facility as able

4. Nutrition Consult to assess adequate intake

DEFINITIONS

ICT-indirect calorimetry testing. Measurement of energy expenditure. This is the most accurate method to determine energy needs. A metabolic cart measures the amount of oxygen consumed and carbon dioxide expired to the amount of oxygen inspired reflecting net substrate utilization. The goal is to improve pulmonary gas exchange and to feed at 100% of REE (resting energy expenditure) to prevent hyperventilation or hypoventilation (excessive removal of carbon dioxide or inadequate removal of carbon dioxide. Check with your respiratory team for a complete listing of guidelines to assess qualifications for your patients. They must meet various qualifications including Fi02 (fraction of inspired oxygen) and PEEP (positive end expiratory pressure) guidelines.

GCS (Glasgow Coma Scale)- a neurological scale is used to assess levels of consciousness. This is a component of the ICH score. A simple, reliable measure to grade intracerebral hemorrhages and mortality risk.

Enteral Nutrition Pathway for Adults

Guidelines for Delivery

Continuous over 24 hrs

Begin at 10-20 mL/hr (especially in ICU or with concentrated formula)

Advance 10 mL every 8-12 hrs to goal rate

Formulas >1.2 Kcal/mL should be started slower and advanced more slowly

Max rate=120 mL/hr for post pyloric feedings

Nocturnal or Cyclic- given continuously at night to increase appetite during the day or to augment PO intake

May wish to provide 50% of needs through TF until pt is able to eat 50-75% of meals. Max rate=120 mL/hr for post pyloric feedings

Bolus/intermittent

**not recommended for PEJ, NJ tubes or post pyloric feeding tube

**not to be use in critically ill patients

Feedings given 3-4 hours a part

If on continuous feedings, hold feedings for 4 hrs prior to first bolus

See attached examples

Post PEG placement- $</=100-120$ mL for first 24 hrs of bolus feeds

<u>Max goal amount is 480 mL per feeding -</u>

<u>240-360 mL per feeding is better tolerated</u>

<u>Especially if you are using a two calorie formula</u>

Gavity feeds- for pt's who are unable to tolerate bolus feedings

Give 120-240 mL over 10 minutes via gravity bag and wait>10 minutes if another bolus is to be given.

It's okay if you only provide 50-75% of estimated needs during the first 24 hrs of bolus feeding. It's better that the pt tolerates the bolus and then advance to ~100% within 2-3 days. Just as you would do with continuous. Goals should never exceed 2 cans at one

time. I usually don't exceed 1.5 cans at one time for individual with caloric needs <2000 Kcals.
Examples for 1.2-1.5 formulas

Bolus tube feeding regimen as follows
(Example of a pt on a goal of 50 mL/hr of continuous feeds)
Flush tube with 30-60 mL of free water pre and post each bolus.
Day one- 120 mL at 9am, 12 noon, 3pm, 6pm, 9pm
Day two-240 mL at 9am, 12 noon, 3pm, 6pm, 9pm (goal) Total of 1200 mL/d

Bolus tube feeding regimen
(Example of a pt on a goal of Continuous feeds of 65 m/hr)
Flush tube with 30-60 mL of free water pre and post each bolus.
Day one- 120 mL at 7am ,10am, 1pm, 4pm, 7pm, 10pm
Day two-220 mL at 7am ,10am, 1pm, 4pm, 7pm, 10pm
Day three-260 mL at 7am ,10am, 1pm, 4pm, 7pm, 10pm (goal) Total of 1560 mL/d

Bolus tube feeding regimen
(Example of a pt on a goal of Continuous feeds of 70 m/hr)
Flush tube with 30-60 mL of free water pre and post each bolus.
Day one- 120 mL at 7am ,10am, 1pm, 4pm, 7pm, 10pm
Day two-220 mL at 7am ,10am, 1pm, 4pm, 7pm, 10pm

Day three-280 mL at 7am ,10am, 1pm, 4pm, 7pm, 10pm (goal) Total of 1680 mL/d

2.0 calorie formula (always start with </=100 mL bolus- do not exceed for 1st 24 hrs secondary to concentration) Pt likely not to tolerate and refuse feedings

(Example of a pt on a goal of Continuous feeds of 40 m/hr)
Start- Day one -100 mL 7am ,10am, 1pm, 4pm, 7pm, 10pm
Day two-160 mL six times daily at 7am ,10am, 1pm, 4pm, 7pm, 10pm (goal) Total of 960 mL/d (1920 Kcals)
Flush tube with 60 mL of free water pre and post each bolus

(Example of a pt on a goal of Continuous feeds of 50 m/hr)
Start- Day one -100 mL 7am ,10am, 1pm, 4pm, 7pm, 10pm
Day two-200 mL six times daily at 7am ,10am, 1pm, 4pm, 7pm, 10pm (goal)
Total of 1200 mL/d (2400 Kcals)
Flush tube with 60 mL of free water pre and post each bolus

Aries Ford, RDN, LDN is a dietitian, motivational speaker specializing in nutrition conferences and workshops. Aries has over 17 years of experience as a dietitian in planning, implementing and coordinating clinical patient nutritional care to promote health and control various diseases. Additional experience includes but not limited to: Nutrition Support Dietitian, total management of parenteral nutrition, Neuroscience Critical care, Gastroenterology and Nephrology. Aries is a graduate of the University of North Carolina at Greensboro and a Buffalo NY native. Aries also enjoys traveling, engaging in media appearances and embracing motherhood of two handsome boys.

Recommended Readings and References

- *Society of Critical Care Medicine (SCCM) and American Society for Parenteral and Enteral Nutrition (ASPEN).JPEN J Parenter/Enteral Nutr.2009:33(3):277-316*
- *Guidelines for the Provision and Assessment of Nutrition Support Therapy in the Adult Critically Ill Patient: Society of Critical Care Medicine*
- *(SCCM) and American Society for Parenteral and Enteral Nutrition (ASPEN)*
- *Society for Parenteral and Enteral Nutrition†. JPEN J Parenter Enteral Nutr published online 15 January 2016.*
- *JPEN J Parenter Enteral Nutr. 2006 Mar-Apr;30(2):71-5*
- *Journal of Neurosurgery Feb.2004/vol.100/No 2:pages 266-271*
- *Vol 67/No 5-pag 668-676*
- *Neurology December 2, 2008 vol. 71 no. 23 1856-1861*

VISIT ARIESFORD.ORG
for more information and a complete listing of other publications

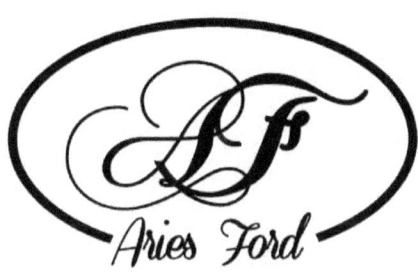

www.ingramcontent.com/pod-product-compliance
Lightning Source LLC
Chambersburg PA
CBHW070430190526
45169CB00003B/1487